Eulogies

When

Christmas

Becomes A Time Of

Loss And Grief:

Writing Guidelines, Examples And Templates

With Tips For Grieving, Healing And Moving On

J Jordan

Notable+

Copyright & Disclaimer

Contents

Preface

Firstly, please accept my deepest condolences. Losing a loved one is an incredibly challenging experience, and I sincerely pray that you find the strength to endure during this time of immense pain and loss.

Loss And Grief At Christmas

Losing a loved one during the holiday season can be an incredibly challenging experience. While the world around us is adorned with festive decorations and filled with joyous celebrations, our hearts may be burdened with grief.

During this time, it is important to find solace and a sense of connection by honoring the memory of our loved ones. One powerful way to pay tribute to their life and legacy is through the art of delivering a eulogy. Not only does a eulogy allow us to express our grief and emotions, but it also provides an opportunity to share cherished memories and celebrate the unique qualities of our loved one.

The Purpose Of This Book

The Christmas season can intensify feelings of grief and loss, making it crucial to strike a balance between honoring the memory of our loved one and participating in the holiday traditions that bring us joy. To assist in navigating this delicate balance, we provide effective strategies for coping with grief during the Christmas season. Furthermore, we delve into the benefits of therapy as a means to cope with grief during this time, offering valuable insights and guidance.

Within the pages of this book, we address the multitude of challenges that arise when writing a eulogy for someone who loved and/or passed away during Christmas. We provide heartfelt eulogy examples and a step-by-step guide to assist you in crafting and delivering a truly meaningful eulogy. In addition, we provide comprehensive answers to commonly asked questions that cover a wide range of topics, such as crafting and organizing the eulogy, handling cherished memories, navigating through grief, and facilitating the healing process.

This book has been meticulously crafted to equip you with the essential tools for navigating the process of writing and delivering a eulogy, all while managing the overwhelming emotions that come with such a difficult period. Our ultimate objective is not only to assist you in creating and delivering a eulogy that truly honors the departed, but also to empower you to navigate the stages of grief and ultimately find solace, healing, and the strength to move forward.

In Difficulty You Are Strengthened

When news of the passing of a loved one arrives, and you find yourself overwhelmed with emotions while simultaneously planning the funeral and holding the rest of the family together, writing a eulogy becomes an arduous task. The raw and gut-wrenching thoughts of your loved one being gone make it challenging to create a eulogy that truly honors their memory. Moreover, amidst all the chaos, you must gather the courage to stand before a grieving audience, paying tribute to the deceased and offering words of encouragement to those in mourning. The weight of this responsibility can feel like an additional burden atop the mountain of challenges you already face.

However, it is a task that must be undertaken, and if you are reading this, it means that this great responsibility has been entrusted to you. I have personally experienced the position you find yourself in right now, and I wholeheartedly empathize with your situation. Despite the overwhelming emotions you may be experiencing, I firmly believe that you possess bravery and courage, even if you may not feel it at this moment.

About Eulogies

The eulogy is a unique and distinct type of speech that requires a different approach due to many factors, including the mental and emotional state of the audience. This book is specifically designed to assist you in this particular task. It is not a generic speech writing guide, as that is not what you need at this moment. My intention is not to delve into the mechanics of speech writing, but rather to provide you with specific wording, examples and templates that you can adapt, replicate and use to craft your tribute or at least inspire and guide your eulogy writing process.

The body of the eulogy contains crucial sections that we have provided for your convenience. These sections can be customized to suit your specific requirements. Within the eulogies presented in this book, you will find introductions, conclusions, and segments dedicated to sharing cherished memories, highlighting the deceased's passions, discussing their influence, and offering words of comfort to those attending the funeral.

Eulogies employ specific language and sections that enable us to effectively convey the sentiments we wish to express. During challenging times, it can be difficult to find the right words and establish a structure that effectively communicates our emotions while paying tribute to someone who held great significance in our lives.

This book also serves as a guide to help you navigate the grieving process while providing examples and templates for eulogy writing. You can largely copy, modify, and adapt these resources to suit the eulogy you are preparing. Its purpose is to alleviate some of the difficulties associated with this task during such a challenging time.

While these eulogies can serve as sources of inspiration, it is important to personalize your tribute to reflect the unique life and relationship you shared with your loved one. Use the structure and themes highlighted here as guides, but make sure to incorporate your own memories, anecdotes, and emotions to create a heartfelt eulogy that truly honors your loved one.

About Sections, Fields, FAQ and More

Eulogy Sections

This book offers a variety of sections that you can customize and incorporate into your eulogy. The language used in these sections is in line with the common expressions found in eulogies. By eliminating the need to fret over the wording or search for the perfect phrases to express your emotions, writing eulogies becomes a less daunting task.

Fields

We have incorporated specific fields, such as [Name], to conveniently accommodate the inclusion of relevant information about the departed individual. These fields greatly assist in tailoring the eulogies to honor your loved one in a personalized manner.

Tips
Italicized tips are a valuable component designed to ignite creativity and motivation within your writing endeavors. These carefully curated suggestions serve as a catalyst for inspiration, encouraging innovative thinking and the exploration of new ideas.

Prompts
These words serve as a compass for your writing endeavors, urging you to include captivating stories, cherished memories, and entertaining anecdotes.

FAQ
Our Frequently Asked Questions (FAQ) section provides comprehensive answers to common inquiries regarding writing eulogies, as well as coping with loss, healing, and moving forward.

Once again, we extend our deepest condolences to you and your loved ones during this time of need. We sincerely pray that you find the strength to carry on.

1. Honoring A Loved One Lost During Christmas

1.1 The Significance Of Remembering And Honoring A Loved One Lost During Christmas

1.1.1 Acknowledging The Pain Of Loss During The Holiday Season

The holiday season is a time of joy, love, and celebration, but for those who have experienced the loss of a loved one, it can also be a poignant reminder of their absence. Christmas, in particular, holds a special place in our hearts, filled with cherished memories and laughter shared with those we hold dear. However, amidst the festivities, it is crucial to acknowledge the pain and grief that accompany the holiday season for those who are mourning. This chapter explores the significance of remembering and honoring a loved one lost during Christmas, offering guidance on reflecting on memories, coping with grief, creating rituals, finding support, embracing emotions, giving back, and finding ways to move forward while still honoring the memory of our beloved departed.

1.1.2 Why It's Important To Remember And Honor Loved Ones During Christmas

Amidst the hustle and bustle of the holiday season, it's crucial to take a moment to pause and remember those who are no longer with us. Honoring their memory is not only an act of love and respect, but it also allows us to keep their spirit alive, even in their absence. By remembering our loved ones, we embrace both the joyful memories they left behind and the impact they had on our lives.

1.2 Reflecting On Memories: Cherishing The Laughter And Joyful Moments Shared

1.2.1 Recalling Special Christmas Memories With A Loved One

The holiday season is a time imbued with nostalgia, and what better way to honor a loved one than by revisiting the cherished memories created together during past Christmases? Whether it's that time they dressed up as Santa Claus and got stuck in the chimney, or the annual family game night that always ended in raucous laughter, these memories bring us comfort and remind us of the joy they brought into our lives.

1.2.2 Embracing The Joyous Moments And Laughter Shared Together

Laughter truly is the best medicine, and during Christmas, we can find solace in reliving the moments of pure joy we shared with our departed loved ones. Embrace the silly traditions, the inside jokes, and the infectious laughter that once filled the room. Share stories with family and friends, and allow yourself to find laughter even in the midst of grieving. It's a beautiful way to honor the memory of someone who brought so much merriment into our lives.

1.3 Coping With Grief: Understanding The Challenges Of Grieving During The Holiday Season

1.3.1 Navigating The Complex Emotions Of Grief During Christmas Time

Grief has this uncanny ability to intensify during the holiday season. The constant reminders of family gatherings and traditions can serve as painful triggers, making it challenging to navigate this often overwhelming emotional journey. It's important to remember that it's okay to feel a whirlwind of emotions – from sadness to anger to even moments of happiness. Give yourself permission to grieve in your own unique way.

1.3.2 Recognizing The Unique Challenges And Triggers Of Grief During The Holiday Season

The holiday season comes with a plethora of potential triggers that can catch us off guard and bring our grief to the forefront. From decorating the Christmas tree to hearing a beloved carol, these seemingly innocent traditions can suddenly become bittersweet reminders of the absence we feel. Understanding and acknowledging these triggers can help us prepare for them and find healthy ways to cope and honor our loved ones amidst the pain.

1.4 Establishing Meaningful Traditions To Honor The Memory Of A Loved One

1.4.1 Developing Personal Rituals To Remember And Honor A Loved One During Christmas

One beautiful way to honor a loved one during the holidays is by creating personal rituals that pay tribute to their memory. Light a candle in their honor, hang a special ornament on the tree, or prepare their favorite dish to share with friends and family. These small but heartfelt gestures create a sense of connection, keeping their spirit alive and reminding us that they are always with us in spirit.

1.4.2 Incorporating The Lost Loved One's Favorite Traditions Into Christmas Celebrations

Another meaningful way to remember a loved one is by incorporating their favorite traditions into our Christmas celebrations. Did they have a favorite holiday movie? Make it a yearly tradition to watch it together. Did they love baking? Whip up a batch of their signature cookies and share them with loved ones. By carrying on these cherished traditions, we not only honor their memory but also find comfort in keeping a piece of them alive in our holiday festivities.

Remember, while the holiday season can be difficult when a loved one is no longer with us, it is also a time when we can come together, share our memories, and find solace in the love that still surrounds us. By embracing the laughter and tears, we can create a meaningful holiday season that honors the memory of those we hold dear.

1.5 Finding Support: Connecting With Others Who Have Experienced Loss During Christmas

1.5.1 Seeking Comfort And Understanding From Support Groups Or Grief Communities

Losing a loved one during Christmas can make this festive season a challenging time. However, finding support and connection with others who have experienced similar losses can provide immense comfort. Support groups and grief communities are excellent resources for navigating the difficult emotions that arise during this time.

Sharing our stories and experiences with individuals who truly understand our pain can be incredibly healing. In these groups, we can openly express our grief, frustration, and even anger, without fear of judgment. Surrounding ourselves with people who have walked the same path helps us feel less alone and validates our emotions.

1.5.2 The Importance Of Sharing Experiences With Others Who Share Similar Losses

When we share our experiences and stories with others who have lost loved ones during Christmas, we create a powerful bond. These connections allow us to commemorate our loved ones together, remembering the laughter and sharing the tears. By sharing our fondest memories, we keep their spirit alive and honor their presence during the holiday season.

Through these connections, we discover that grief is a universal experience and that we can find solace in knowing we are not alone. By listening to others' stories, we may even find inspiration and hope for our own healing journey. Building relationships with others who have experienced similar losses can help us navigate the holiday season with a renewed sense of support.

1.6 Allowing Space For Sadness During The Holiday Season

1.6.1 Validating And Accepting The Tears And Sadness That May Arise During Christmas

Amidst the festivities, it is essential to remember that it's okay to feel sad during Christmas after losing a loved one. Grief doesn't take a holiday, and it's important to validate our feelings of sadness. Instead of trying to suppress or ignore these emotions, we must embrace them and allow ourselves the space to mourn.

By acknowledging and accepting our tears, we honor the depth of our love for our departed loved one. It is a testament to the special connection we shared and the impact they had on our lives. We should never feel ashamed or inadequate for experiencing sadness during the holidays; it is a natural part of the grieving process.

1.6.2 Finding Healthy Ways To Cope With Grief And Emotions During The Holiday Season

While it's crucial to embrace our sadness, it's equally vital to find healthy coping mechanisms for managing grief during the holiday season. Engaging in activities that bring us comfort and solace can help us navigate the emotional rollercoaster that Christmas can bring.

This may involve engaging in self-care practices such as exercise, meditation, or journaling. It could also mean seeking professional counseling or therapy to receive guidance in processing our emotions. Finding healthy outlets like these allows us to balance our grief with a glimmer of joy and aids in our healing process.

1.7 Engaging In Acts Of Kindness And Charity In Memory Of A Loved One

1.7.1 Paying Tribute By Volunteering Or Donating To Causes That Were Important To The Lost Loved One

A beautiful way to honor the memory of a loved one during Christmas is by engaging in acts of kindness and charity. Many lost loved ones held causes close to their hearts, and by volunteering or donating to those causes, we pay tribute to their legacy.

Whether it's supporting a charity, participating in a fundraising event, or volunteering our time, these gestures of goodwill allow us to carry on their spirit. By giving back, we create a positive impact on the world, and in turn, find solace and purpose in our grief journey.

1.7.2 Spreading Love And Kindness During The Holiday Season In Honor Of The Person We Have Lost

In addition to supporting causes dear to our loved ones, we can also spread love and kindness in their memory. Simple acts of compassion, such as reaching out to those who may be feeling lonely or extending a helping hand to those in need, can make a significant difference during the holiday season.

By embodying the values our loved ones cherished, we honor their memory and make the world a little brighter. Spreading love and kindness not only benefits others but also brings comfort and meaning to our own hearts during a time of grief.

1.8 Creating New Traditions: Honoring The Memory Of A Loved One While Embracing The Present

1.8.1 Incorporating Special Rituals Or Activities That Remind Us Of Our Loved One During Christmas

As we navigate the first Christmas without our loved one, it can be comforting to incorporate special rituals or activities that remind us of them. Setting a place at the table for them, lighting a candle, or playing their favorite holiday music are beautiful ways to include their presence in our celebrations.

By intentionally integrating these traditions, we keep our loved one's memory alive and create a space for them at our holiday gatherings. These small gestures help us feel connected to our departed loved one, allowing their spirit to be a part of our holiday festivities.

1.8.2 Balancing Grief And Joy By Creating New Traditions That Bring Happiness And Comfort

While it is essential to honor our loved one's memory, it is equally important to create new traditions that bring us joy and comfort. Christmas can still hold a place for happiness amidst the grief. This might involve trying out new holiday recipes, exploring different decorations, or engaging in activities that bring us genuine happiness.

Finding a delicate balance between remembering our loved one and embracing the present allows us to navigate Christmas with a renewed sense of hope. By creating new traditions, we adapt to our evolving lives while keeping our departed loved one close to our hearts.

As we navigate the holiday season without our loved ones, it is important to remember that it is okay to feel a mix of emotions, from laughter to tears. By cherishing the memories, establishing meaningful rituals, finding support from others who understand, and giving back in their honor, we can find solace and strength during this time.

Though their physical presence may be missed, the love and laughter they brought into our lives will forever remain in our hearts. May we find comfort in knowing that by honoring their memory, we continue to keep their spirit alive. Let us remember the laughter, share the tears, and carry their love with us always.

2. Eulogies When Christmas Becomes A Time Of Loss And Grief

2.1 Navigating Loss And Grief During The Holiday Season

2.1.1 The Unique Challenges Of Grieving During Holidays

For those who have experienced the loss of a loved one during the holiday season, it can be an emotionally challenging and overwhelming time. Dealing with grief during holidays poses unique difficulties, as traditional festivities and gatherings can serve as painful reminders of the absence of those we hold dear. In this chapter, we will explore the complexities of navigating loss and grief during the holiday season, and provide insights and strategies to help individuals not only cope with their emotions but also find ways to honor and remember their loved ones while seeking healing and hope.

2.2 Acknowledging And Validating Emotions: The Importance Of Grieving During Holidays

2.2.1 Allowing Yourself To Feel: Embracing The Full Range Of Emotions

During the holiday season, it's common to feel a mix of emotions including sadness, anger, and nostalgia. It's vital to give yourself permission to experience these emotions and not suppress them. Allow yourself to cry, reminisce, or simply take a moment to acknowledge your feelings. By embracing the full range of emotions, you give yourself the space to heal and honor your grief.

2.2.2 Normalizing Grief: Understanding That It's Okay To Grieve During Holidays

It's also important to remember that grieving during the holidays is completely normal. Society often puts pressure on us to be cheerful and merry, but grief doesn't adhere to a holiday schedule. It's okay to feel sad when everyone else seems to be jolly. Your grief is valid, and it's important to remind yourself that you don't have to put on a happy face just because it's the holiday season.

2.3 Finding Support: Building A Network Of Understanding And Compassionate Individuals

2.3.1 Reaching Out For Support: Identifying Trusted Friends And Family

During times of grief, having a support system can make a world of difference. Reach out to friends and family members who you feel comfortable talking to about your feelings. Share your experiences and allow them to support you in whatever way feels right for you. Sometimes, just knowing that you're not alone can bring immense comfort.

2.3.2 Joining Support Groups Or Therapy: Professional Help For Coping With Grief

If you find that you need additional support, consider joining a support group or seeking therapy. These can provide a safe space to share your feelings and connect with others who are going through similar experiences. Having a professional guide you through your grief can be incredibly helpful in finding healthy coping mechanisms and navigating the complex emotions that arise during the holidays.

2.4 Honoring And Remembering: Creating Meaningful Rituals And Traditions

2.4.1 Designing Personal Rituals: Expressing Love And Remembrance

In the midst of grief, finding ways to honor and remember your loved ones or the loss you've experienced can bring a sense of comfort and connection. Consider creating personal rituals that allow you to express your love, such as lighting a candle, visiting a special place, or writing a letter. These rituals can be tailored to your unique relationship with the person or the significance of the loss.

2.4.2 Incorporating The Memory Of Loved Ones: Including Their Presence In Holiday Celebrations

Additionally, finding ways to incorporate the memory of your loved ones into holiday celebrations can help keep their presence alive. Whether it's hanging a photo ornament on the tree, sharing stories of their favorite holiday traditions, or setting a place at the table in their honor, these gestures can bring a sense of warmth and inclusion during what may otherwise feel like an empty time.

Remember, grieving during the holidays is a personal journey, and there is no right or wrong way to navigate it. Trust yourself, be kind to yourself, and give yourself permission to grieve in whatever way feels authentic to you.

2.5 Self-Care During The Holidays: Strategies For Coping With Grief And Loss

2.5.1 Practicing Self-Compassion: Granting Yourself Grace And Understanding

Losing a loved one can make the holiday season especially challenging. It's crucial to remember to take care of yourself during this time. Practicing self-compassion is essential. Allow yourself to grieve and feel whatever emotions come up, without judgment. Grant yourself grace and understanding, knowing that it's okay to not feel joyous during a time that emphasizes happiness. Give yourself permission to take breaks and prioritize your emotional well-being.

2.5.2 Maintaining Healthy Boundaries: Prioritizing Your Well-Being

During the holiday season, it's common for others to try to include you in activities and celebrations. While it's important to connect with loved ones, it's equally important to maintain healthy boundaries. Be honest with yourself about what you can handle and communicate your needs to others. Don't be afraid to decline invitations or modify plans to suit your emotional needs. Prioritize your well-being and ensure you're setting aside time for self-care.

2.6 Re-Evaluating Expectations: Adjusting Holiday Plans And Priorities

2.6.1 Setting Realistic Expectations: Redefining The Meaning Of Holiday Celebrations

Grief can change the way we approach the holiday season. It's essential to re-evaluate our expectations and redefine the meaning of holiday celebrations. Instead of trying to recreate past traditions, consider creating new ones or modifying existing ones to honor your loved one's memory. Embrace the idea that the holidays may look different now, and that's okay. By setting realistic expectations and focusing on meaningful moments, you can find comfort and solace during this time.

2.6.2 Finding Comfort In Simplicity: Scaling Down Traditions And Activities

The holiday season often comes with a whirlwind of activities and obligations. However, when grieving, it may be helpful to scale down and simplify. Focus on what brings you the most comfort and joy, and let go of the rest. It's okay to say no to certain events or traditions that feel overwhelming. Embrace the simplicity of the moment and find solace in quieter, more reflective activities that allow you to honor your loved one's memory in a meaningful way.

2.7 Supporting Others: How To Offer Comfort And Understanding To Those Grieving

2.7.1 Being Present And Available: Providing A Safe Space For Expression

If you have loved ones who are grieving during the holidays, it's important to offer your support. One of the best ways to do this is by being present and available. Create a safe space for them to express their emotions openly without judgment. Be a listening ear and a shoulder to lean on. Your presence and willingness to be there for them during this difficult time can make a world of difference.

2.7.2 Showing Empathy And Compassion: Offering Practical Support And Listening

In addition to being present, it's crucial to show empathy and compassion when supporting others who are grieving. Understand that grief is a unique and ongoing process, and everyone experiences it differently. Offer practical support, whether it's helping with daily tasks, cooking a meal, or running errands. Most importantly, be a compassionate listener and avoid pressuring them to "move on" or "cheer up." Allow them to share their memories and feelings, and offer your support in whatever way they need.

2.8 Moving Forward: Finding Hope And Healing After Loss During The Holidays

2.8.1 Finding Meaning And Purpose: Creating A Sense Of Renewal

While grief can feel overwhelming, it's possible to find hope and healing during the holiday season.

One way to do this is by finding meaning and purpose in your grieving journey. Consider engaging in activities that honor your loved one's memory, such as volunteering or starting a new tradition that brings you joy. By finding ways to create a sense of renewal and connection, you can find solace in knowing that your loved one's legacy lives on.

2.8.2 Focusing On The Future: Embracing Hope And Building Resilience

Lastly, it's important to focus on the future and embrace hope. Grief doesn't mean forgetting or letting go; it means finding a way to move forward while cherishing the memories. Use this time to build resilience and discover new possibilities in your life. Surround yourself with supportive people, seek professional help if needed, and believe in your ability to heal and find joy again. By embracing hope and focusing on the future, you can navigate through grief and find moments of happiness even during the holiday season.

While the holiday season can be a difficult time when grieving, it is essential to remember that it is okay to feel a mix of emotions. By acknowledging and validating these emotions, seeking support from understanding individuals, and creating meaningful rituals and traditions, it is possible to find comfort and healing during this challenging period. By practicing self-care, re-evaluating expectations, and offering support to others, we can navigate the holiday season with compassion and empathy. Remember, healing takes time, and it is important to be patient and kind to ourselves as we move forward. May the holidays become a time of reflection, remembrance, and finding hope for the future.

3. Honoring The Memory Of A Loved One Through A Holiday Eulogy

3.1 The Power Of A Holiday Eulogy

Honoring the memory of a loved one is an important part of the grieving process, and finding meaningful ways to remember them is deeply personal. One powerful way to commemorate their life and keep their spirit alive is through a holiday eulogy. This chapter explores the significance of delivering a eulogy during a holiday, providing a platform to reflect on the life and legacy of your loved one. Through this heartfelt tribute, you can share memories, celebrate their impact, and find solace in the healing power of honoring their memory during a time of togetherness and remembrance. Discover how to craft a meaningful holiday eulogy that brings comfort, healing, and a sense of connection to both yourself and those who gather to remember your loved one.

3.2 Reflecting On The Life And Legacy Of Your Loved One

3.2.1 Embracing The Grief And Healing Process

Losing a loved one is an incredibly challenging experience, and navigating through grief is a personal journey. Embracing the grief and healing process is an important step in preparing to create a holiday eulogy. Take the time to acknowledge your emotions, seek support from loved ones or a support group, and allow yourself to grieve in your own way. By embracing the healing process, you can better honor your loved one's memory and create a eulogy that truly reflects their impact on your life.

3.2.2 Identifying Key Aspects Of Your Loved One's Life

When reflecting on the life and legacy of your loved one, it's important to identify key aspects that made them who they were. Consider their passions, accomplishments, values, and unique qualities that set them apart. Were they known for their sense of humor, their unwavering kindness, or their dedication to a cause? By pinpointing these key aspects, you can weave them into your eulogy and create a heartfelt tribute that captures the essence of your loved one.

3.3 Crafting A Meaningful And Heartfelt Eulogy

3.3.1 Understanding The Purpose And Structure Of A Eulogy

Crafting a eulogy requires careful thought and planning. Begin by understanding the purpose and structure of a eulogy. A eulogy is a tribute that captures the essence of a person's life, highlighting their accomplishments, qualities, and impact on others. It typically includes an introduction, personal anecdotes and stories, reflections on their character and values, and a conclusion that leaves a lasting impression. By understanding the purpose and structure, you can organize your thoughts and create a eulogy that flows naturally and resonates with the audience.

3.3.2 Honoring The Unique Qualities And Contributions Of Your Loved One

In crafting a holiday eulogy, it's essential to honor the unique qualities and contributions of your loved one. Share stories and anecdotes that exemplify their character and values. Highlight their passions, accomplishments, and the impact they had on others' lives. Remember to incorporate their sense of humor, their wisdom, or any other qualities that made them special. By celebrating the individuality of your loved one, you create a eulogy that is both meaningful and a genuine reflection of the person they were.

As you embark on the journey of creating a holiday eulogy, remember that this is an opportunity to both grieve and celebrate the life of your loved one. Share your emotions, memories, and stories with sincerity and let their spirit shine through your words. By embracing the power of a holiday eulogy, you can create a lasting tribute that not only honors their memory but also brings comfort and connection during the holiday season.

3.4 Sharing Memories And Stories To Celebrate Your Loved One

The holiday season is a time for bringing people together, and what better way to honor the memory of a loved one than by sharing cherished stories and memories? Collecting and organizing meaningful anecdotes and memories can be a heartwarming and cathartic process.

3.4.1 Collecting And Organizing Meaningful Anecdotes And Memories

Gather your family and friends and create a space to reminisce about your loved one. Share stories that capture their essence and bring back fond memories. These stories can be anything from heartwarming moments to funny anecdotes that depict their unique personality. Consider reaching out to loved ones who may have their own special memories to share. Collating these stories will help you create a rich tapestry of your loved one's life.

To organize these memories, consider creating a chronological timeline or grouping them by themes that resonate with your loved one's passions and interests. By putting these memories in order, you can ensure a coherent and meaningful eulogy that truly captures their spirit.

3.4.2 Highlighting The Impact And Influence Of Your Loved One

In addition to sharing stories, it's important to highlight the impact and influence your loved one had on others. Were they a mentor, a healer, a pillar of strength, or a source of inspiration? Reflect on the ways in which they touched the lives of those around them. By highlighting their positive contributions, you are not only celebrating their memory but also reminding everyone of the lasting impact they had on the world.

3.5 Incorporating Rituals And Symbolism Into The Eulogy

Incorporating rituals and symbolism into the eulogy can provide a powerful sense of connection and remembrance. It allows you to honor your loved one's beliefs, values, and traditions.

3.5.1 Exploring Symbolic Gestures And Traditions

Consider incorporating symbolic gestures or traditions that held significance for your loved one. This could include lighting a candle in their memory, playing their favorite song, or sharing a special recipe that was a holiday tradition. These small acts can serve as poignant reminders of their presence and the love you shared.

3.5.2 Creating A Sacred Space For Remembrance And Connection

To create a sacred space for remembrance and connection, you can decorate a special area with items that hold meaning for your loved one. This could be a table adorned with photographs, mementos, or objects that represent their passions and interests. By having this space, you provide both yourself and others with a physical reminder of their life and the love that surrounds them.

3.6 Supporting And Including Family And Friends In The Eulogy

The grieving process is not something that should be done alone. Involving family and friends in the eulogy can provide support and create a sense of unity as you honor your loved one.

3.6.1 Collaborating And Gathering Contributions From Loved Ones

Reach out to family members and close friends to gather their thoughts, memories, and reflections. Their contributions can add depth and variety to the eulogy, allowing for a more comprehensive portrait of your loved one. By including multiple perspectives, you create a collective tribute that celebrates their life from different angles.

3.6.2 Honoring Relationships And Acknowledging Support Networks

Acknowledge the relationships your loved one had with others and the support networks that surrounded them. Take the time to mention and thank those who provided comfort and assistance during difficult times. By recognizing the importance of connections, you not only pay homage to your loved one but also demonstrate the power of love and community.

3.7 Embracing Healing Through A Holiday Eulogy

Writing a holiday eulogy not only honors the memory of your loved one but also provides an opportunity for healing and remembrance. By sharing stories, incorporating rituals and symbolism, and involving family and friends, you create a heartfelt tribute that celebrates their life and legacy. Embrace this process as a way to find solace and joy in the midst of grief and to keep their spirit alive during the holiday season.

In times of loss, a holiday eulogy can provide a powerful opportunity to pay tribute to our loved ones. By reflecting on their life and sharing heartfelt memories, we can find solace, healing, and a renewed sense of connection. Whether it's through storytelling, incorporating rituals, or involving family and friends, a holiday eulogy allows us to embrace the healing process, keep the spirit of our loved ones alive and find solace during times of mourning.

4. Crafting The Eulogy: A Step-By-Step Guide To Writing A Meaningful Tribute

4.1 Understanding The Purpose And Structure Of A Eulogy

A eulogy serves as a heartfelt tribute to the person who has passed away. It's an opportunity to reflect on their life, share memories, and celebrate their accomplishments. Understanding the purpose of a eulogy is key to crafting a meaningful tribute.

The structure of a eulogy typically includes an introduction, where you establish your connection to the person and set the tone for the speech. Then, you can delve into different aspects of their life – childhood, achievements, relationships, and so on. Finally, conclude the eulogy by summarizing the impact they had on others and expressing gratitude for the time shared together.

4.2 Gathering Information And Personal Reflections

When writing a eulogy, it's helpful to gather information from various sources: family members, friends, colleagues, and even the person's own writings or speeches. Listen to the stories and anecdotes they share, and reflect on your own personal experiences with the individual.

Take time to recollect specific moments, conversations, or actions that truly exemplify who they were. These personal reflections will add depth and authenticity to your eulogy. Remember, it's not just about listing achievements or accolades – it's about capturing the essence of the person and sharing it with others.

4.3 Organizing And Crafting The Eulogy With Care

With the gathered information and personal reflections in hand, it's time to organize and craft your eulogy. Begin by creating an outline, highlighting the key themes or aspects you want to cover. Then, fill in the details and connect them in a way that flows naturally.

While it's important to be concise, don't be afraid to inject humor or share personal anecdotes that will resonate with the audience. You want the eulogy to feel authentic and true to the person you are honoring. Remember, it's not about impressing others with your writing skills; it's about expressing genuine emotions and capturing the essence of the person's life.

4.4 Leaving A Lasting Legacy And Finding Closure

4.4.1 Reflecting On The Individual's Impact And Legacy

As you bring your eulogy to a close, take a moment to reflect on the person's impact and legacy. Consider the ways in which they touched the lives of others, the positive change they brought to their community, and the lasting memories they created.

Their legacy is not just about the achievements or titles they held, but about the lasting impressions they made on the hearts and minds of those they encountered. By honoring and acknowledging this impact, you help to ensure that their memory lives on.

4.4.2 Finding Closure And Moving Forward With Inspiration

Writing and delivering a eulogy is a cathartic process that allows us to find closure and begin the healing journey. As you conclude your eulogy, remember to offer words of comfort and strength to those in attendance. Share your own commitment to carry forward the values and lessons learned from the person you've lost, finding inspiration in their life to guide you on your own path.

Though the journey may be bittersweet, by celebrating a life full of purpose and passion, we can find solace in knowing that our loved one's memory will continue to inspire us and others for years to come.

4.5 A Celebration Of Life

As we conclude the journey of celebrating a life full of purpose and passion, be reminded of the profound impact one individual can have on the world. Through the process of writing a eulogy, we honor their accomplishments, share cherished memories, and embrace the emotions that come with loss. By delivering a heartfelt tribute, we ensure that their legacy lives on, inspiring others to follow their example of living with purpose and passion. May this act of remembrance bring us closure, while reminding us to seize each day with intention and make a difference in the lives of those around us.

5. Delivering The Eulogy: Tips For Public Speaking And Connecting With The Audience

5.1 Preparing For The Emotional Challenge Of Public Speaking

Public speaking can be an emotional challenge, especially when delivering a eulogy. Take the time to prepare yourself mentally and emotionally before stepping up to the podium. Practice reading the eulogy out loud, allowing yourself to become comfortable with the words and emotions associated with them.

If you feel overwhelmed during the delivery, take deep breaths and remind yourself of the love and admiration you have for the person you are honoring. Embrace the vulnerability of the moment, knowing that sharing your feelings will help others in their own grieving process.

5.2 Engaging The Audience And Establishing A Connection

When delivering a eulogy, it's important to establish a connection with the audience. Speak from the heart, make eye contact, and use body language to convey your emotions. Engage the audience by sharing relatable stories or inviting them to participate in a moment of reflection or remembrance.

Remember, the eulogy is not just for you—it's an opportunity to bring people together, to uplift their spirits, and to honor the person's memory as a collective group. By creating a sense of connection, you can help others find solace, inspiration, and comfort during this difficult time.

5.3 Leaving A Lasting Legacy Through Words

Crafting and delivering a meaningful eulogy is an opportunity to leave a lasting legacy for your loved one. By choosing your words carefully and sharing heartfelt sentiments, you can honor their life and create a lasting impact on those who hear your tribute. Remember that the power of a eulogy lies not only in the memories it evokes but also in the comfort and solace it provides to those who are grieving. Embrace this chance to celebrate a life well-lived and give your loved one a meaningful send-off.

6. Eulogy Examples And Templates

The holiday season is a time of immense joy and celebration, but it can also serve as a poignant reminder of those we have lost. It is during this time that we seek solace and a sense of connection by honoring the memory of our loved ones. One profound way to pay tribute to their life and enduring legacy is through the delivery of a holiday eulogy. This heartfelt gesture not only allows us to express our grief and emotions, but also presents an opportunity to share cherished memories and celebrate the unique qualities that made our loved ones so special.

Within this section, we present four poignant eulogies that serve as a testament to the lives of those who departed during the Christmas season or held a deep affection for this cherished holiday. Each eulogy has been carefully divided into specific components, each contributing to the creation of a well-crafted eulogy. You can include any or all of the components, depending on your personal preferences and the circumstances surrounding your situation. Feel empowered to edit and adapt these templates as you see fit, incorporating your own experiences, stories, and quotes into the appropriate sections.

May these eulogies serve as a guiding light for those who find themselves faced with the daunting task of crafting and delivering a eulogy for a departed loved one, particularly during the season of Christmas. May you find solace and strength to endure this period of loss.

7. Eulogy 1 - An Inspiring Eulogy Dedicated To Our Mother, Who Passed Away On Christmas Day

7.1 Remembering Our Guardian Angel

7.1.1 Introductions And Greetings

In the depths of grief, we gather here today to pay tribute to our beloved mother, who was not only our guiding light but also our guardian angel. I am [Your Name], [Name]'s [Your relationship to the deceased] and I am honored to speak on behalf of the loved ones gathered here today. With heavy hearts and tearful eyes, we celebrate the life of our dear mother, who departed from this world on a day eternally intertwined with love and joy - Christmas Day. As we navigate the journey of honoring her memory, we find solace in the cherished moments and profound impact she had on our lives. This eulogy serves as a heartfelt remembrance, a testament to the beautiful soul that continues to watch over us, inspiring us with her love, resilience, and unwavering presence.

7.1.2 The Loved Ones Who Continue The Legacy

Our beloved [Name]'s passing has left a profound void in our lives. In reflecting on [her] life, it is important to acknowledge those who continue to carry on [her] legacy. [Name] is survived by [State and name the close kins e.g.{ [her] loving family, including [her] devoted [spouse], [Name] and their [number] children [List Names], who were the center of [her] universe.]} [State and name other relatives e.g.{ [She] leave(s) behind a host of cherished relatives, including nieces, nephews, and cousins whom [she] held dear.]} Additionally, [she] touched the lives of countless friends and acquaintances through [her] graciousness and unwavering support. [Her] presence will be greatly missed by all who had the privilege of knowing [her]. Despite the immense sorrow that accompanies this loss, we take comfort in the knowledge that [Name] has left an indelible mark on the lives of those whom [she] graciously touched with love and joy.

7.1.3 A Life Well-Lived: Introducing Our Mother's Journey

To truly honor the memory of our beloved mother, we must take a moment to reflect on the incredible life she lived. From her humble beginnings to the person she became, our mother's journey was filled with triumphs and setbacks, laughter and tears. She faced challenges head-on, turning her dreams into reality and leaving an indelible mark on everyone she encountered.

7.1.4 The Impact Of Losing Our Guardian Angel

Losing our mother on Christmas Day is a heart-wrenching blow that words can hardly capture. She was not only our parent but also our confidante, guiding us through life's maze with unwavering love and support. Her absence leaves a void that can never be filled, but we find solace in knowing that she will forever remain our guardian angel, watching over us from above.

7.2 Cherished Memories: Celebrating Our Mother's Life

7.2.1 Childhood Adventures: Recalling Joyful Moments With Our Mother

As children, our mother was the mastermind behind countless adventures that filled our hearts with joy. From spontaneous road trips to impromptu picnics in the park, she taught us the value of seizing the moment and finding happiness in the simplest of pleasures. These cherished memories will forever bring a smile to our faces and warmth to our hearts.

[**Prompt:** Include stories of your mother and her teachings from your childhood.]

7.2.2 Unconditional Love: How Our Mother Nurtured And Supported Us

Our mother's love knew no bounds. She was our biggest cheerleader, always there to uplift us during both triumphs and tribulations. Her unwavering support and nurturing nature provided us with the strength to chase our dreams and conquer our fears. We carry her love within us, a beacon of light guiding us through life's uncertainties.

[**Prompt:** Share stories of your mother's support and how it impacted your life.]

7.2.3 Shared Traditions: Keeping Our Mother's Legacy Alive

One of the many legacies our mother leaves behind is the traditions she instilled in us. Whether it was baking cookies on Christmas Eve or Sunday family gatherings, these rituals were the threads that bound our family together. Though her physical presence may be gone, we honor her memory by carrying on these cherished traditions and keeping the flame of love and togetherness burning.

[**Prompt:** Share stories of your mother's Christmas traditions and how it impacted your life.]

7.3 A Loving Support System: Our Mother's Role As Our Guardian Angel

7.3.1 A Pillar Of Strength: How Our Mother Guided And Protected Us

In times of uncertainty and hardship, our mother was our rock, providing unwavering guidance and protection. She had a unique ability to navigate the stormiest seas of life, offering us a steady hand to hold onto. Her strength became our strength, empowering us to face life's challenges with courage and determination.

7.3.2 Selfless Sacrifices: Remembering The Ways Our Mother Always Put Us First

Our mother's selflessness knew no bounds. She always put our needs before her own, sacrificing her time, energy, and desires to ensure our well-being and happiness. Her acts of love and sacrifice serve as a constant reminder of the incredible person she was, and we strive to emulate her example of putting others first.

7.4 Lessons Of Love And Resilience: The Impact Our Mother Had On Our Lives

7.4.1 Life Lessons Learned: The Teachings Our Mother Instilled In Us

Our mother was not just a source of love and support but also a wise teacher. She imparted invaluable life lessons that continue to shape us into the individuals we are today. From teaching us the importance of kindness and empathy to instilling the value of hard work and perseverance, her teachings serve as guiding principles that will forever help us navigate life's winding path.

7.4.2 Overcoming Challenges: Drawing Inspiration From Our Mother's Resilience

Our mother faced numerous challenges throughout her life, and it was her resilience that inspired us all. She taught us that setbacks are not the end but rather opportunities for growth. Her unwavering determination in the face of adversity serves as a constant reminder that we, too, can overcome any obstacle. Her spirit lives on within us, pushing us to face the world head-on with unwavering resolve.

7.4.3 Cherishing The Memories And Impact Of Our Guardian Angel

In our hearts, our mother will forever be our guardian angel, guiding and protecting us from above. Her life may have passed, but her impact will forever remain etched in our souls. We will carry her love, strength, and wisdom with us always, honoring her memory by living the extraordinary lives she believed we could lead.

7.5 Embracing Her Legacy: Carrying Forward Our Mother's Values And Beliefs

Losing someone dear is heartbreaking. But as we come to terms with the void left by our beloved mother, we find solace in knowing that her legacy lives on through us. Our mother was a woman of strong values and unwavering beliefs, and it is our duty to embody her spirit and keep her memory alive.

7.5.1 Embodying Her Spirit: How We Honor Our Mother's Core Values

Our mother taught us the importance of kindness, compassion, and empathy. In her honor, we strive to treat others with the same warmth and understanding that she showed to everyone she encountered. Whether it's lending a listening ear, offering a helping hand, or spreading love throughout our community, we honor her by embracing the values she instilled in us.

7.5.2 Paying It Forward: Continuing Our Mother's Acts Of Kindness

[Name] had a heart full of generosity and a passion for helping those in need. To honor her memory, we have taken it upon ourselves to continue her acts of kindness. We volunteer at local charities, donate to causes close to her heart, and seek opportunities to make a positive impact, just as she did. By carrying forward her altruistic spirit, we ensure that her legacy of compassion lives on.

7.6 Finding Solace: Coping With The Loss Of Our Guardian Angel

Grief is a complex journey, and navigating it can be overwhelming. But as we grieve the loss of our guardian angel, we find comfort in coming together as a family. We support one another, allowing ourselves the space to process our emotions and heal together.

7.6.1 Navigating Grief: Processing Our Emotions And Healing Together

The loss of our mother has brought waves of sorrow, but we have realized that grief is not something to be endured alone. We openly share our feelings, our tears, and our memories, finding solace in knowing that we have each other to lean on. By acknowledging our emotions and allowing ourselves to mourn, we take the necessary steps towards healing and finding peace.

7.6.2 Finding Comfort: Honoring Our Mother's Memory Through Rituals And Reflection

In the midst of grief, we have found solace in honoring our [Name]'s memory through rituals and reflection. We gather on special occasions to recount cherished memories, light a candle in her honor, or simply spend time reminiscing about the beautiful moments we shared. These acts bring us closer to her spirit, allowing us to find comfort in the presence of her memory.

7.7 Christmas Day Remembrance: Honoring Our Mother's Spirit On This Special Day

Losing our mother on Christmas Day is a bittersweet reminder of the profound impact she had on our lives. While the holiday season may bring a mix of emotions, we have found ways to honor her spirit and keep her memory alive during this time of year.

7.7.1 A Bittersweet Celebration: How We Remember Our Mother During Christmas

Christmas was [Name]'s favorite time of year, filled with joy, love, and the joyous sounds of laughter. Though her absence is deeply felt, we celebrate Christmas in her honor, embracing the traditions she held dear. We cherish the memories of decorating the tree together, singing carols, and sharing heartfelt moments of togetherness.

7.7.2 Creating New Traditions: Incorporating Our Mother's Presence Into The Festivities

In addition to continuing our mother's cherished traditions, we have also found solace in creating new ones that incorporate her presence. Whether it's preparing her favorite holiday dishes, setting a place at the table in her memory, or playing her favorite Christmas songs, these heartfelt gestures help us feel closer to her spirit, ensuring that she remains an integral part of our celebrations.

7.8 Conclusion: Cherishing The Memories And Impact Of Our Guardian Angel

7.8.1 The Enduring Impact Of Our Amazing Mother

Though our [Name] may no longer be physically with us, her love and guidance will forever remain in our hearts. We are eternally grateful for the gift of having her as our guardian angel, and we carry her memory forward with love and admiration. As we embrace her values, find solace in togetherness, and honor her during special occasions, we keep her spirit alive and ensure that her impact on our lives will never fade.

7.8.2 Forever Grateful For Our Guardian Angel's Love And Guidance

As we conclude this tribute to our guardian angel, we are filled with a profound sense of gratitude for the love and guidance our dear mother bestowed upon us. Though [Name]'s physical presence may be absent, her spirit remains alive within each of us, guiding our steps and filling our hearts with warmth. We vow to carry forward her legacy, cherishing the memories and embracing the values she instilled in us. Our mother's love will forever be a beacon of light in our lives, and as we navigate the days ahead, we find comfort in knowing that she watches over us from heaven. Farewell, dear guardian angel, until we meet again.

8. Eulogy 2 - A Eulogy For My Beloved Father Who Passed Away During Christmas

8.1. Introduction: Remembering The Life Of My Beloved Father

8.1.1 A Heartfelt Tribute: Honoring The Life And Legacy

Losing someone we love is never easy, especially when it happens during a time that is meant for joy and celebration. I am [Your Name], [Name]'s [son/daughter] and I am honored to speak on behalf of the loved ones gathered to remember and pay tribute to the life of my beloved father, who left us unexpectedly during the Christmas season. Although his departure has left a void in our hearts, we choose to focus on the beautiful memories and the positive impact he had on our lives. Let us come together to pay tribute to a man who touched the lives of many and left an indelible mark on this world.

8.1.2 The Loved Ones Who Continue The Legacy

Our beloved [Name]'s passing has left a profound void in our lives. In reflecting on [his] life, it is important to acknowledge those who continue to carry on [his] legacy. [Name] is survived by [State and name the close kins e.g. {[his] loving family, including [his] devoted [wife/spouse], [Name] and their [number] children [List Names], who were the center of [his] universe.]} [State and name other relatives e.g. {[He] leave(s) behind a host of cherished relatives, including nieces, nephews, and cousins whom [he] held dear.]} Additionally, [he] touched the lives of countless friends and acquaintances through [his] graciousness and unwavering support. [His] presence will be greatly missed by all who had the privilege of knowing [him]. Although this loss brings immeasurable grief, we find solace in knowing that [Name] has engendered a lasting impact on those whose lives [he] gracefully enhanced with love and joy.

8.1.3 A Time Of Reflection: Embracing The Grieving Process

Grief is a complex journey that we must navigate in our own unique ways. As we gather here today, it is important to acknowledge that each one of us is experiencing this loss differently. Let us embrace this time of reflection and support one another as we mourn the passing of our dear [Name]. Together, we can find solace in shared memories, laughter, and tears. In the face of loss, we find strength in unity and comfort in the love we have for [Name].

8.2 A Life Well-Lived: Celebrating His Accomplishments And Contributions

8.2.1 A Man Of Integrity: Examining His Professional Achievements

My father was a man of unwavering integrity and dedication. Throughout his professional career, he achieved great things and earned the respect of his colleagues and peers. From his unmatched work ethic to his innovative ideas, he left an undeniable impact in his field. His achievements serve as a reminder that success is not solely measured by accolades, but by the mark we leave on the lives of others.

8.2.2 A Giving Soul: Remembering His Philanthropic Endeavors

In addition to his professional accomplishments, [Name] was a beacon of generosity. He believed in the power of giving back to the community and selflessly dedicated his time and resources to various philanthropic causes. Whether it was volunteering at local charities or supporting organizations close to his heart, his compassion knew no bounds. Today, we celebrate his legacy of kindness and the countless lives he touched through his selflessness.

[**Prompt:** Give specific examples of the deceased's support to philanthropic causes.]

8.3 Cherishing The Bond Between Father And Child

8.3.1 A Role Model And Mentor: Lessons Learned From A Father's Love

As a father, my dad was not just a provider but also a guiding light in my life. He taught me invaluable lessons about love, compassion, and resilience. His unwavering support and belief in my abilities shaped me into the person I am today. My father's unconditional love and unwavering guidance will forever be a reminder of the importance of family and the profound impact a parent can have on their child's life.

[**Prompt:** Give an example of one of the deceased's lessons that you were taught]

8.3.2 Shared Memories: The Special Moments And Traditions We Shared

Beyond the life lessons, my father and I shared countless precious memories together. From our annual family vacations to simple moments spent laughing around the dinner table, those cherished times will forever hold a special place in my heart. The Christmas traditions we created, the jokes we shared, and the love we showered upon each other are memories that I will treasure for a lifetime. Although he may no longer be physically with us, his spirit and the bond we shared will endure.

[**Prompt:** Give a story, memory or Christmas tradition that you and your loved one shared.]

8.4 Lessons In Resilience: Reflecting On The Strength And Determination He Showed

8.4.1 Overcoming Challenges: Stories Of Triumph And Perseverance

Life is not without its challenges, and my father faced his fair share. Yet, he demonstrated remarkable resilience and determination in overcoming those hurdles. His ability to rise above adversity inspired all who knew him, reminding us that setbacks are merely stepping stones on the path to success. In the face of difficulties, he showed us the importance of maintaining a positive outlook and never giving up.

8.4.2 Inspiring Others: How His Resilience Continues To Impact Lives

Even though my father is no longer here, his resilience continues to inspire and impact the lives of those who knew him. Through his example, he taught us the importance of perseverance, the strength of the human spirit, and the ability to find light even in the darkest of times. As we honor his memory, let us carry forward his legacy by embodying the qualities he stood for – resilience, determination, and the unwavering belief that we can overcome whatever challenges life throws our way.

8.5 Spreading Joy: Recalling The Happy Memories And Laughter He Brought

8.5.1 The Lighter Side: Fond Memories Of His Sense Of Humor

When I think back on my beloved father, one word immediately comes to mind: laughter. He had an uncanny ability to lighten the mood and bring a smile to everyone's face. Whether it was his cheesy dad jokes or his hilarious dance moves at family gatherings, he knew exactly how to make us laugh. I'll never forget the times we spent doubled over in laughter, tears streaming down our faces, thanks to his quick wit and infectious humor. Those memories will forever hold a special place in my heart.

[**Prompt:** Give an example of your lovedones's sense of humor by sharing a funny story or a joke of his.]

8.5.2 Creating Happiness: Celebrating The Joys He Brought Into Our Lives

Beyond making us laugh, my father was a master at creating happiness, especially during Christmas. He was the person who could turn any ordinary day into a celebration. From surprise ice cream trips to impromptu dance parties in the living room, he knew how to make even the simplest moments feel special. He taught us the importance of finding joy in the little things and embracing the present moment. The legacy of happiness he leaves behind is something that I will always strive to carry forward in my own life.

8.6 Healing Through Grief: Coping Strategies And Support In Times Of Loss

8.6.1 Navigating The Emotional Rollercoaster: Understanding The Stages Of Grief

Losing a loved one during the holiday season can be particularly difficult. While the world around us is filled with festive decorations and joyous celebrations, our hearts may be heavy with grief, and navigating the various emotions that come with grief can feel like riding a rollercoaster. It's important to recognize and understand the stages of grief: denial, anger, bargaining, depression, and acceptance. Remember, there is no right or wrong way to grieve, and it's okay to experience a wide range of emotions. Allow yourself to feel and process your grief in your own time and seek support from loved ones or professionals who can guide you through this difficult journey.

8.6.2 Finding Solace: Coping Mechanisms And Seeking Support

While grief is unique to each individual, there are coping mechanisms that can help ease the pain. Engaging in self-care activities like journaling, exercising, or spending time in nature can provide solace and a sense of grounding during this challenging time. It's important to find a balance between honoring the memory of our loved one and allowing ourselves to participate in the holiday traditions that bring us joy. Additionally, seeking support from friends, family, or support groups can provide a safe space to share your feelings and receive comfort from those who understand your loss. Remember, healing takes time, so be patient with yourself and allow yourself to grieve in your own way.

8.7 Legacy And Remembrance: Honoring His Memory And Carrying On His Spirit

As we reflect on the life of my beloved father, it's essential to focus on the legacy he leaves behind. His impact on our lives will forever be cherished and remembered. Whether it's through sharing stories, preserving his favorite recipes, or continuing his acts of kindness, we have the power to carry on his spirit. We can honor his memory by living our lives with the same love, laughter, and joy that he brought into our lives. While [Name] may no longer be physically with us, his presence will always remain alive in our hearts and in the way we choose to live our lives.

As I conclude this eulogy for my beloved father, I am reminded of his immense love, strength, and the lasting impact he had on my life and the lives of those around him. While his physical presence may be gone, his spirit and teachings will forever guide and inspire me. As we honor his memory and carry his legacy forward, let us remember the joy he brought, the lessons he imparted, and the love he shared. May his spirit continue to shine brightly, not just during Christmas, but each and every day of our lives.

9. Eulogy 3 - Finding Solace In The Season: A Eulogy For Our Christmas-Loving Hero

9.1 Remembering Our Christmas-Loving Hero

9.1.1 Introduction And Greeting

In a world that sometimes feels dark and chaotic, there are those rare individuals who possess a special gift. Our Christmas-loving hero was one such person. [He/She/They] lived and breathed the holiday spirit, finding solace and joy in the magic that Christmas brought. I am [Your Name], [Name]'s [Your relationship to the deceased] and I am honored to speak on behalf of the loved ones gathered here today to remember this remarkable individual who taught us the true meaning of the season and left an indelible mark on our hearts.

9.1.2 The Loved Ones Who Continue The Legacy

Our beloved [Name]'s passing has left a profound void in our lives. In reflecting on [his/her/their] life, it is important to acknowledge those who continue to carry on [his/her/their] legacy. [Name] is survived by [State and name the close kins e.g.{ [his/her/their] loving family, including [his/her/their] devoted [husband/wife/spouse], [Name] and their [number] children [List Names], who were the center of [his/her/their] universe.]} [State and name other relatives e.g.{ [He/She/They] leave(s) behind a host of cherished relatives, including nieces, nephews, and cousins whom [he/she/they] held dear.]} Additionally, [he/she/they] touched the lives of countless friends and acquaintances through [his/her/their] graciousness and unwavering support. [His/Her/Their] presence will be greatly missed by all who had the privilege of knowing [him/her/them]. In the face of this immense sorrow that has befallen us, we seek solace in the profound realization that [Name] has left an indelible mark on the lives of those fortunate enough to have encountered [his/her/their] limitless love and contagious joy.

9.2 A Life Embraced By The Magic Of Christmas

9.2.1 Early Memories: Our Hero's First Encounters With Christmas

From a young age, [Name] was captivated by the wonder and enchantment that filled the air during the Christmas season. [His/Her/Their] eyes sparkled with delight as [he/she/they] eagerly awaited the arrival of Santa Claus, clutching an ever-growing list of wishes. The magic of decorating the Christmas tree, hanging stockings by the fireplace, and opening presents on that special morning filled [his/her/their] heart with glee.

9.2.2 Creating A Winter Wonderland: Decorating With Enthusiasm

No other pursuit brought [Name] as much joy as adorning [his/her/their] home in a festive spectacle. From the roof to the front yard, the house became an oasis of twinkling lights, reindeer figures, and inflatable snowmen. Passersby would stop in awe, marveling at the dedication and creativity that went into transforming a simple dwelling into a winter wonderland. [Name]'s enthusiasm for decorating was infectious, inspiring others to embrace their own holiday spirit.

9.3 The Power Of Tradition: Creating Beloved Memories

9.3.1 Family Traditions: Our Hero's Commitment To Rituals

[Name] understood the power of tradition in bringing loved ones closer together. Each year, [he/she/they] meticulously planned activities and rituals that would create lasting memories for the family. From baking gingerbread cookies and watching classic holiday movies to singing carols around the piano, our hero ensured that these traditions were cherished and passed down through generations. [He/She/They] knew that the true magic of Christmas resided in the love and togetherness shared with family.

9.3.2 Community Involvement: Spreading Christmas Cheer Beyond The Home

But our hero's love for Christmas was not confined to [his/her/their] own household; [he/she/they] extended [his/her/their] joy and kindness to the wider community. Whether it was volunteering at local charities, organizing toy drives, or attending neighborhood Christmas festivities, our hero believed in sharing the holiday spirit with everyone [he/she/they] encountered. [Name]'s commitment to spreading joy and cheer was a testament to [his/her/their] generous heart and the belief that Christmas had the power to unite and uplift.

[**Prompt:** Include a memory or story of your loved one sharing the holiday spirit with others.]

9.4 Spreading Joy And Kindness: Our Hero's Acts Of Christmas Generosity

9.4.1 Secret Santa Surprises: Touching Lives With Anonymous Gifts

[Name] had a mischievous side, too. [He/She/They] embraced the spirit of Secret Santa with gusto, secretly leaving unexpected gifts for friends, colleagues, and even strangers. These acts of anonymous kindness brought smiles to faces and warmth to hearts, reminding us all of the magic that can be found in simple acts of giving.

[**Prompt:** Share a personal example of your loved one's mischievous and fun side.]

9.4.2 Charitable Initiatives: Our Hero's Impact On Those In Need

[Name]'s love for Christmas extended far beyond the exchange of presents. [He/She/They] recognized that some in our community were less fortunate and in need of assistance during the holiday season. With unwavering compassion, our hero spearheaded charitable initiatives to bring joy and relief to those facing hardship. Whether it was organizing food drives, raising funds for shelters, or personally delivering gifts to children in need, our hero's impact on the lives they touched was immeasurable.

[**Prompt:** Share specific examples of your loved one supporting others in need.]

9.5 Battling Grief: Finding Comfort In The Holiday Season

The holiday season can be a bittersweet time for those who have suffered the loss of a loved one. The twinkling lights, familiar carols, and aroma of gingerbread can amplify the void left by our departed Christmas-loving hero. However, amidst the grief, there are coping strategies that can help us navigate the pain of loss during this time.

9.5.1 Coping Strategies: Navigating The Pain Of Loss During Christmas

Finding solace during the holiday season starts with acknowledging our emotions. It's okay to feel sadness, nostalgia, and even anger. Remember that grief is a personal journey, and everyone experiences it differently. Allow yourself to grieve and heal in your own time and in your own way.

9.5.2 Reaching Out For Support

Reach out for support during this time. Share your feelings with friends and family who can provide a listening ear and a comforting shoulder. Joining support groups, whether online or in person, can also connect you with others who understand the unique challenges of grieving during the holidays.

9.5.3 Incorporating Self-Care

Self-care becomes particularly important during this difficult period. Give yourself permission to take breaks when needed, indulge in activities that bring you joy, and take care of your physical and mental well-being. Remember, it's not selfish to prioritize self-care during a time of mourning.

9.6 Celebrating Memories: Incorporating Our Hero's Presence In Holiday Traditions

One way to honor our Christmas-loving hero and find comfort is by incorporating [his/her/their] presence in our holiday traditions. Set a special place at the dinner table, hang a cherished ornament on the tree, or light a candle in [his/her/their] memory. By including our hero in these traditions, we keep [Name]'s spirit alive and feel [his/her/their] love and joy in the midst of our grief.

9.6.1 Sharing Stories And Memories

Sharing stories and memories of our hero can also be a meaningful way to celebrate [his/her/their] life. Collecting anecdotes from family and friends and creating a memory jar or a photo album can remind us of the happiness [he/she/they] brought into our lives. These shared moments can become cherished traditions that help us connect with our hero's spirit during the holiday season.

9.6.2 Passing Down Traditions: Ensuring Christmas Spirit Lives On

[Name]'s love for Christmas was infectious, and it's important to keep that spirit alive. Passing down traditions [he/she/they] cherished, whether it's baking [his/her/their] favorite Christmas cookies or watching beloved holiday movies, helps us connect with [his/her/their] joyous energy. By involving future generations in these traditions, we ensure that the magic of Christmas lives on in our family for years to come.

9.7 Embracing The Spirit Of Christmas: Lessons Learned From Our Hero

Our Christmas-loving hero taught us valuable lessons about embracing the true spirit of the holiday season. As we mourn [Name]'s loss, we can honor [his/her/their] memory by incorporating these lessons into our own lives.

9.7.1 Finding Joy In Small Moments: Emulating Our Hero's Appreciation For The Season

[Name] showed us how to find joy in the simple pleasures of the holiday season. From savoring a steaming cup of hot cocoa to getting lost in the beauty of twinkling lights, we can follow in [his/her/their] footsteps and embrace the magic that surrounds us. Let's take a moment to slow down, appreciate the small things, and find happiness in the enchantment of the season, just as our hero did.

9.7.2 Spreading Love And Kindness: Incorporating Our Hero's Values Into Everyday Life

[Name]'s love for Christmas was not just about the decorations and festivities; it was about spreading love and kindness. Let's carry that torch forward by volunteering our time, donating to those in need, and offering a helping hand to those who are struggling. By incorporating our hero's values into our everyday lives, we can continue to make the world a brighter, more compassionate place, not just during the holiday season, but all year round.

9.8 Conclusion: Celebrating The Life And Love Of Our Beloved

While grief may cast a shadow during the holiday season, it's important to remember that the love [Name] brought into our lives will forever burn bright. We are filled with gratitude for the joy [he/she/they] brought into our lives. [His/Her/Their] unwavering spirit, acts of kindness, and dedication to keeping the magic of Christmas alive will forever remain in our hearts. May [his.her/their] memory continue to inspire us to cherish the holiday season and the precious moments we share with loved ones. Though [Name] is no longer physically with us, [his/her/their] love for Christmas will forever shine brightly, guiding us through the darkest of times. [Name]'s love for Christmas lives on, reminding us that the magic of the season can be found in the warmth of our hearts and in the love we share with others.

10. Eulogy 4 - A Eulogy For A Loved One Who Died At Christmas Time

10.1 Introduction: Welcome Greetings

Ladies and gentlemen, family and friends, thank you all for gathering here today, though the circumstances that bring us together are undoubtedly somber. Today, we gather not only to mourn the passing of our beloved [Name] but to celebrate the beautiful life that touched each and every one of us in profound ways. I am [Your Name], [Name]'s [Your relationship to the deceased] and I am honored to speak on behalf of the loved ones gathered here today.

10.2 The Loved Ones Who Continue The Legacy

Our beloved [Name]'s passing has left a profound void in our lives. In reflecting on [his/her/their] life, it is important to acknowledge those who continue to carry on [his/her/their] legacy. [Name] is survived by [State and name the close kins e.g.{ [his/her/their] loving family, including [his/her/their] devoted [husband/wife/spouse],

[Name] and their [number] children [List Names], who were the center of [his/her/their] universe.]} [State and name other relatives e.g.{ [He/She/They] leave(s) behind a host of cherished relatives, including nieces, nephews, and cousins whom [he/she/they] held dear.]} Additionally, [he/she/they] touched the lives of countless friends and acquaintances through [his/her/their] graciousness and unwavering support. [His/Her/Their] presence will be greatly missed by all who had the privilege of knowing [him/her/them]. Even though this loss brings us immeasurable sadness, we take comfort in the knowledge that [Name] has left a lasting impact on the lives of those whom [he/she/their] lovingly touched with joy and happiness.

10.3 Acknowledging Grief During Christmas

It is with heavy hearts that we say our goodbyes during this Christmas season, a time typically reserved for joy, laughter, and togetherness. Yet, in the midst of our collective grief, let us remember the extraordinary person we are here to honor.

[Name] was a light in our lives, a beacon of warmth and kindness that brightened even the darkest of days. [His/Her/Their] departure at this time of year serves as a poignant reminder of the fragility of life and the bittersweet nature of our existence.

10.4 Remembering The Deceased's Love For Christmas

During the holiday season, [Name] not only embraced the festive spirit with enthusiasm but also infused it with [his/her/their] own special magic. [His/Her/Their] generosity knew no bounds, and the joy [he/she/they] spread was infectious. Christmas was not just a season for [him/her/them]; it was a philosophy, a way of being that centered around love, compassion, and selflessness.

10.5 Cherishing Memories

As we reflect on the memories we shared with [Name], let us focus not only on the sorrow of [his/her/their] absence but on the profound impact [he/she/they] had on each of us. [He/She/They] leaves behind a legacy of love, kindness, and a deep sense of connection.

10.6 Continuing The Legacy Of Love

[Name]'s spirit will forever live on in the twinkling lights, the laughter of children, and the warmth of shared moments. In our grief, let us find solace in the knowledge that [he/she/they] would want us to continue spreading love and joy, just as [he/she/they] did during countless holiday seasons.

10.7 The Lessons We Carry

Let us carry the lessons of [Name]'s life with us as we navigate the challenges of the coming days, weeks, and years. May [his/her/their] memory be a guiding light, inspiring us to be better, to love more deeply, and to cherish the moments we have with those we hold dear.

10.8 Conclusion: Reflection And Saying Goodbye

In this time of sorrow, let us lean on each other for support and find comfort in the shared memories that bind us together. As we say our goodbyes, let us remember [Name] not with tears of sadness but with smiles that reflect the love [he/she/they] brought into our lives.

While [Name] may no longer be physically present, [his/her/their] legacy can continue to shine brightly during the holiday season.

Rest in peace, dear [Name], and may the angels sing you to your eternal rest. You will be deeply missed, especially during this season of love and joy.

11. Finding Peace And Healing Amidst Yuletide Sorrow

11.1 Understanding Yuletide Sorrow And Its Impact

The holiday season, often associated with joy, warmth, and celebration, can also be a challenging time for those experiencing grief and loss. Yuletide sorrow, as we refer to it, encompasses the complex emotions that arise when mourning intersects with the festivities of this time of year. Whether it's the absence of a loved one, the heaviness of past traumas, or the feeling of being overwhelmed by the expectations of the season, Yuletide sorrow weighs on the hearts of many. In this chapter, we explore the impact of grief during the holidays and provide insights and strategies to navigate this difficult journey. By acknowledging and honoring our emotions, embracing self-care, seeking support, and finding new ways to celebrate and remember, we can discover moments of peace and healing amidst the Yuletide sorrow.

11.1.1 What Is Yuletide Sorrow?

Yuletide Sorrow is like the Grinch that sneaks into our hearts during the holiday season. It's that overwhelming feeling of sadness, grief, and loss that can hit us harder than Mariah Carey hitting those high notes in "All I Want for Christmas." While everyone else is decking the halls and fa-la-la-ing, those experiencing Yuletide Sorrow may find it challenging to muster up the holiday cheer.

11.1.2 The Emotional Toll Of Grieving During The Holidays

Grief is tough enough on any regular day, but throwing in tinsel, twinkling lights, and jolly tunes can make it feel like a festive slap in the face. The holiday season magnifies our emotions, and for those mourning the loss of a loved one or going through a difficult time, it can be an emotional rollercoaster. The sight of a beautifully wrapped gift may trigger memories of our dearly departed or highlight the absence of someone we hold dear. It's a tough reality to face when everyone else seems to be singing carols and guzzling eggnog without a care in the world.

11.2 Navigating Grief During The Holiday Season

11.2.1 Recognizing And Validating Your Emotions

First things first, it's essential to recognize and acknowledge that it's okay to feel sad during the holidays. Your emotions are valid, and you don't have to force yourself into fake smiles and fake holiday spirit. Give yourself permission to grieve, cry, and feel whatever you need to feel. It's your emotional journey, and you're the one in control of your own sleigh.

11.2.2 Coping Strategies For Dealing With Grief

Finding healthy coping strategies can be key to navigating the holiday season with Yuletide Sorrow. Whether it's journaling your thoughts, indulging in warm bubble baths, or binging on your favorite holiday movies, find what brings you comfort and peace. And don't forget the sweet power of hot cocoa – it's like a warm hug from the inside.

11.2.3 Setting Boundaries: Communicating Your Needs To Others

Remember, you're the boss of your emotions, and nobody can dictate how you should feel or act during this time. Don't be afraid to set boundaries and communicate your needs to your friends and family. Let them know that while you appreciate their love and support, you may need some space or understanding during this season. It's like a polite way of saying, "Please, keep the reindeer games to yourselves."

11.3 Embracing Self-Care: Healing Practices For Yuletide Sorrow

11.3.1 Practicing Self-Compassion And Self-Forgiveness

During times of grief, it's crucial to practice self-compassion and cut yourself some slack. Give yourself permission to take a step back from the expectations and pressures of the holiday season. Remember, you're doing the best you can, and that's more than enough. If you accidentally burn the Christmas cookies or forget to send out holiday cards, give yourself a break. Santa's got nothing on your self-love.

11.3.2 Utilizing Relaxation Techniques For Stress Reduction

Stress and grief go together like mistletoe and awkward office parties. That's why incorporating relaxation techniques into your routine can be a game-changer. Whether it's deep breathing exercises, meditation, or simply taking a long, peaceful walk in the snow (or sand, depending on where you are), find moments of calm amidst the chaos. Trust us; it's like finding a quiet spot in a crowded shopping mall – a rare and precious gem.

11.3.3 Engaging In Physical Activities To Promote Well-Being

Channel your inner Rudolph and get moving! Physical activities not only boost your endorphin levels but can also help distract your mind from the sorrow. Whether it's lifting weights, going for a jog in the winter wonderland, or busting out some epic dance moves to "Jingle Bell Rock," find what gets your body moving and your spirits grooving.

11.4 Seeking Support: Connecting With Loved Ones And Communities

11.4.1 Reaching Out To Friends And Family For Emotional Support

Your friends and family may not be mind readers, but they're pretty darn close when it comes to supporting you. Don't hesitate to lean on those who care about you during this time. Share your feelings, memories, or even your favorite ugly Christmas sweater with them. A listening ear, a warm hug, or a shoulder to cry on can make all the difference in the world.

11.4.2 Joining Support Groups Or Therapy For Grief Counseling

Sometimes, our loved ones might not fully understand the depth of our grief. That's when support groups or therapy can step in like Santa's little helpers. Joining others who are going through similar experiences can provide a safe space to share, heal, and find solace. Remember, it takes a village, or in this case, a gingerbread house of supportive individuals, to help us through.

11.4.3 Participating In Community Events And Volunteer Opportunities

If you're ready to step out of your comfort zone, participating in community events or volunteering can help shift your focus and provide a sense of purpose. Spread a little holiday cheer to those who need it most, and you might find that your own heart starts to heal in the process. Plus, who wouldn't want to wear an elf hat while making the world a better place?

Remember, Yuletide Sorrow doesn't have to be a never-ending loop of "Blue Christmas." By recognizing your emotions, taking care of yourself, and seeking support, you can find moments of peace and healing amidst the holiday season. So embrace your journey, hold on to those cherished memories, and know that you're not alone in this snowy adventure.

11.5 Celebrating The Spirit Of Loved Ones During Yuletide

11.5.1 Creating Remembrance Rituals Or Traditions

With the holiday season often bringing a sense of loss and longing, creating remembrance rituals or traditions can help keep the spirit of loved ones alive. Whether it's lighting a candle for them, sharing stories and memories, or even cooking their favorite dish, these small acts can bring comfort and a sense of connection.

11.5.2 Displaying Memorabilia Or Photo Collections

Another way to honor the memory of loved ones is by displaying their memorabilia or photo collections. This can serve as a beautiful reminder of their presence and the impact they had on our lives. It's like having a mini tribute gallery that celebrates their life and keeps their memory close to our hearts.

11.5.3 Writing Letters Or Expressing Gratitude For The Influence Of Loved Ones

Sometimes, the best way to cope with sorrow during the Yuletide season is by expressing our emotions through writing. Taking the time to write a letter to our loved ones, expressing gratitude for the impact they had on our lives, can be incredibly healing. It allows us to acknowledge their presence, even if they are no longer physically with us.

11.6 Creating New Traditions: Finding Meaning And Joy Amidst Sorrow

11.6.1 Exploring Different Ways To Celebrate The Holiday Season

When grief casts a shadow on the holiday season, it might be helpful to explore different ways to celebrate. Maybe this is the year to try new activities or traditions that bring joy and meaning. It could be volunteering at a local shelter, organizing a cozy movie night with friends, or even taking a solo trip to a place that holds special meaning. The key is to listen to our hearts and find what brings us comfort and happiness.

11.6.2 Incorporating Rituals Or Activities That Promote Healing

In the midst of sorrow, it's important to prioritize self-care and healing. Incorporating rituals or activities that promote healing can be incredibly beneficial. This could be anything from practicing mindfulness meditation to attending support groups or therapy sessions. By intentionally making space for healing, we can gradually find solace and peace during the Yuletide season.

11.6.3 Engaging In Acts Of Kindness And Giving Back To Others

Sometimes, finding joy amidst sorrow can come from acts of kindness and giving back to others. Whether it's donating to a local charity, volunteering our time, or simply offering a helping hand to someone in need, these acts bring a sense of purpose and fulfillment. Not only do they bring positivity into the lives of others, but they can also ignite a spark of joy within ourselves.

11.7 Cultivating Mindfulness: Embracing The Present Moment During The Holiday Season

11.7.1 Practicing Mindfulness Meditation And Breathing Exercises

Amidst the chaos and bittersweetness of the holiday season, practicing mindfulness meditation and breathing exercises can help us ground ourselves in the present moment. By bringing our attention to the here and now, we can find moments of peace and clarity. Taking a few minutes each day to tune in to our breath and calm our minds can make a world of difference in navigating the Yuletide season.

11.7.2 Focusing On Gratitude And Appreciation For The Present

In the midst of sorrow, it's easy to get caught up in what's missing or no longer there. However, shifting our focus to gratitude and appreciation for the present can help us find moments of joy. Taking time each day to reflect on the things we are grateful for can bring a renewed sense of hope and warmth, reminding us that there is still goodness to be found, even in difficult times.

11.7.3 Avoiding Comparison And Embracing Imperfections

The holiday season often comes with societal pressures and expectations that can exacerbate feelings of sorrow and inadequacy. It's important to remember that everyone's journey is unique, and it's okay to embrace imperfections. Instead of comparing ourselves to others or chasing an unattainable idea of perfection, let's focus on being kind to ourselves and finding solace in the imperfect beauty of our own experiences.

11.8 Looking Ahead: Hope And Resilience In The New Year

As the Yuletide season comes to a close, it's natural to start looking ahead to the new year. It's a time for reflection, renewal, and setting intentions for the future. Despite the sorrows of the past, let's embrace the hope and resilience that come with a new beginning. By carrying the memories of loved ones in our hearts and nurturing our own well-being, we can face the future with strength and optimism.

In conclusion, while Yuletide sorrow may cast a shadow during the holiday season, it is essential to remember that healing and peace are within reach. By embracing our emotions, practicing self-care, seeking support, honoring memories, creating new traditions, cultivating mindfulness, and holding onto hope, we can find solace amidst the sorrow. Let this time of year be a reminder that healing is a journey, and by taking each step with compassion and resilience, we can navigate the holiday season with grace and find moments of joy and peace along the way.

12. Seeking Professional Help: How Therapy Can Provide Guidance During Hard Holiday Times

12.1 Introduction: A Time Of Celebration And Challenges

12.1.1 Understanding The Challenges Of Holiday Season

The holiday season is often portrayed as a time of joy, togetherness, and celebration. However, for many individuals, this time of year can be incredibly challenging. The pressures of social obligations, financial strain, and heightened expectations can contribute to feelings of stress, anxiety, and sadness. During these hard holiday times, seeking professional help through therapy can provide invaluable guidance and support. This final chapter explores the importance of reaching out for therapeutic assistance during the holiday season, the various types of therapy available, and how therapy can offer strategies to navigate holiday-related stress, grief, and loss. By embracing therapy as a resource during difficult times, individuals can find solace, healing, and hope amidst the holiday chaos.

12.1.2 Recognizing The Emotional Struggles Faced During The Holidays

For many people, this time of year can bring about a range of complex emotions and challenges. From feelings of loneliness and grief to heightened financial stress and family conflicts, the holiday season can intensify pre-existing emotional struggles and create new ones.

12.1.3 The Impact Of Holiday-Related Stress On Mental Health

Holiday-related stress can have a significant impact on our mental health. The pressure to create picture-perfect celebrations, meet societal expectations, and maintain a cheerful facade can be overwhelming. This stress can lead to increased anxiety, depression, and feelings of inadequacy. It's crucial to recognize the toll that holiday-related stress can take on our mental well-being and seek support when needed.

12.2 The Importance Of Seeking Professional Help During Difficult Times

12.2.1 Breaking The Stigma: Acknowledging The Benefits Of Therapy

In times of emotional turmoil, seeking professional help can be a game-changer. Therapy offers a safe and non-judgmental space to explore our emotions, gain insight into ourselves, and develop coping strategies. It's important to break the stigma around therapy and acknowledge that seeking help is a sign of strength, not weakness. Just as we would seek medical help for a physical ailment, seeking therapy for our mental well-being is equally essential.

12.2.2 The Role Of Therapeutic Guidance In Overcoming Holiday Challenges

Therapy provides valuable guidance and support for navigating the challenges that the holiday season brings. A skilled therapist can help us identify and process our emotions, develop healthy coping mechanisms, and set realistic expectations. They can offer fresh perspectives, provide tools for effective communication, and assist in building resilience. With the guidance of a therapist, we can regain a sense of control and find ways to navigate the holidays with greater ease.

12.3 Types Of Therapy: Finding The Right Approach For You

12.3.1 Exploring Different Therapy Approaches And Modalities

Therapy comes in various forms, each tailored to address specific needs and preferences. From traditional talk therapy to more specialized approaches like cognitive-behavioral therapy (CBT) or mindfulness-based therapy, there is a wide range of options to explore. It's essential to find a therapy approach and modality that resonates with you, as this can significantly impact the effectiveness of your therapeutic experience.

12.3.2 Understanding The Potential Benefits Of Individual, Group, And Family Therapy

Individual therapy offers one-on-one sessions with a therapist, allowing for personalized attention and a focus on individual goals. Group therapy provides the opportunity to connect with others going through similar struggles and gain support from peers. Family therapy can help improve communication and understanding within familial relationships. Each type of therapy has its unique benefits, and it's important to choose the one(s) that align with your needs and circumstances.

12.4 How Therapy Can Provide Guidance And Support During The Holidays

12.4.1 Creating A Safe Space For Emotional Expression And Validation

The holiday season can stir up a whirlwind of emotions, and therapy offers a safe space to express and process these feelings. Therapists provide a judgment-free environment where you can openly discuss your fears, frustrations, and sadness without the fear of burdening others. This emotional validation can be incredibly liberating and empowering, allowing you to navigate the holidays with a greater sense of self-awareness and emotional well-being.

12.4.2 The Role Of Therapists In Offering Practical Strategies For Coping With Holiday Stress

Therapists are equipped with a wide range of practical strategies and tools to help you cope with holiday stress. From stress management techniques to boundary-setting skills, therapists can guide you in developing effective coping mechanisms that align with your unique situation. They can help you identify triggers, manage expectations, and create a self-care routine to navigate the holidays in a way that prioritizes your well-being.

Remember, seeking professional help during difficult holiday times is not a sign of weakness, but rather a powerful step towards self-care and growth. A therapist can provide the support, guidance, and tools you need to navigate the holiday season with greater ease and emotional well-being.

12.5 Addressing Holiday-Related Stress And Anxiety In Therapy Sessions

The holiday season is often touted as a time of joy and celebration, but for many, it can also bring a wave of stress and anxiety. From navigating family dynamics to financial pressures and the overwhelming expectations of creating the perfect holiday experience, it's no wonder that this time of year can be particularly challenging for some.

In therapy sessions, one of the first steps is identifying the specific triggers that cause holiday-induced anxiety. Whether it's the fear of disappointing loved ones or the pressure to meet societal standards of holiday cheer, understanding these triggers can help develop strategies for managing and coping with them.

Therapists can offer techniques for stress reduction and emotional well-being during the holidays. From mindfulness exercises to breathing techniques and grounding practices, these tools can help individuals find moments of calm amidst the chaos. By incorporating these techniques into daily routines, clients can build resilience and better navigate the stressors that tend to arise during this time of year.

12.6 Developing Coping Strategies: Techniques Offered By Therapists

While therapy provides a safe space to explore and address holiday-related stress and anxiety, it also offers an opportunity to develop coping strategies that extend beyond the therapy session. Therapists can introduce mindfulness and relaxation techniques as effective tools for holiday stress relief.

Mindfulness exercises, such as meditation or body scans, can help individuals stay present and focused, reducing the tendency to get caught up in the whirlwind of holiday chaos. Relaxation techniques, like deep breathing and progressive muscle relaxation, provide instant relief for heightened stress levels.

Additionally, therapists can help clients build resilience and set realistic expectations for the holiday season. Often, there is a pressure to create picture-perfect moments during the holidays, but this can be an unrealistic and exhausting pursuit. By working with a therapist, individuals can understand and embrace their limitations, setting boundaries and focusing on what truly matters to them.

12.7 Navigating Grief And Loss During The Holiday Season With Therapeutic Support

The holiday season can be especially challenging for those who have experienced the loss of a loved one. Festive times may serve as painful reminders of their absence, intensifying feelings of grief and loneliness. However, therapy can provide valuable support during this difficult period.

Therapists can help clients navigate the complex emotions associated with the loss of a loved one during the holidays. Through compassionate listening and guidance, therapists can assist individuals in finding healthy ways to cope and honor their grief. This may involve developing rituals or engaging in activities that memorialize the deceased, creating space for healing and remembrance.

12.8 Embracing Healing And Hope Through Therapy During Hard Holiday Times

While the holiday season can be a challenging time, therapy offers a beacon of hope and healing. Through addressing holiday-related stress and anxiety, developing coping strategies, and navigating grief and loss, therapists provide crucial support and guidance.

By identifying triggers, managing stress through relaxation techniques, and setting realistic expectations, therapy equips individuals with the tools to approach the holiday season with greater ease and resilience. And for those grappling with grief, therapeutic support can help honor the memory of their loved ones while finding solace amidst the festivities.

Remember, seeking professional help during hard holiday times is not a sign of weakness but rather a brave step towards self-care and emotional well-being. By embracing therapy, individuals can find the support they need to navigate the holiday season with grace, compassion, and maybe even a touch of humor. After all, therapy doesn't have to be all serious; sometimes, a little laughter can lighten the load and remind us that we're all in this holiday chaos together.

By embracing therapy as a resource, individuals can embrace healing, find hope, and reclaim the joy that the holiday season can bring.

Frequently Asked Questions
A. Writing The Eulogy

A.1 Can anyone contribute to the eulogy?

Yes, absolutely. The eulogy is an opportunity for friends, family members, and loved ones to share their personal memories and reflections on the deceased's life. If you would like to contribute to the eulogy, reach out to the person organizing the service or the individual designated to speak during the ceremony.

A.2 How long should the eulogy be?

The length of the eulogy can vary depending on the traditions, preferences, and time constraints of the memorial service. Generally, a eulogy is around 5 to 10 minutes long, allowing enough time to capture the essence of the departed's life and impact. However, it is important to remember that quality matters more than quantity. Focus on sharing meaningful stories and heartfelt messages that truly honor your loved one.

A.3 Can I include humor in the eulogy?

Yes, incorporating lighthearted and humorous anecdotes can be a beautiful way to celebrate the joyful moments and unique personality of the departed. However, it is essential to strike a balance and be mindful of the overall tone of the service. Ensure that any humor is respectful and appropriate for the occasion, keeping in mind the feelings of the grieving family and attendees.

A.4 Is it necessary to follow a particular structure for the eulogy?

While there is no one-size-fits-all structure for a eulogy, it is helpful to have a loose outline to guide your speech. Consider including sections such as an introduction, sharing personal memories, highlighting achievements and contributions, discussing the impact on loved ones, and concluding with a heartfelt farewell. However, feel free to adapt the structure to best reflect the unique life and relationships shared with your loved one.

A.5 How can I structure the eulogy for maximum impact?

To ensure the eulogy resonates with the audience, organizing it in a cohesive and impactful manner is key. Begin with an introduction that captures attention and expresses gratitude for the life of our colleague. Then, progress through personal stories, highlighting their achievements, character traits, and moments that made them special. Conclude with a heartfelt message that leaves the listeners feeling uplifted and motivated to honor their memory.

B. The Eulogy And Coping With Loss At Christmas

B.1 How can crafting a heartfelt eulogy help in coping with the loss during the holiday season?

Writing and delivering a heartfelt eulogy provides an opportunity to reflect on the life and legacy of your beloved family member. It allows you to honor their memory, share cherished memories and stories, and find comfort in celebrating their life amidst the holiday season. Crafting a eulogy can be a cathartic process that promotes healing and helps in navigating through grief during this time.

B.2 How can we keep the Christmas spirit alive while grieving the loss of our loved one?

Keeping the Christmas spirit alive while grieving involves finding solace in cherished traditions shared with your loved one. Engaging in acts of kindness, generosity, and spreading love can help honor their memory. It's important to seek support from family and friends, embrace the symbolism of Christmas, and draw strength from faith and spirituality to find comfort during this difficult time.

B.3 How can we include our departed loved one in Christmas celebrations without feeling overwhelmed by grief?

Including your departed loved one in Christmas celebrations can be a way of keeping their memory alive. You can incorporate their favorite traditions, prepare their beloved dishes, or create a special memorial ornament in their honor. It's important to set boundaries and allow yourself to feel emotions, while also finding moments of joy and connection with others. Remember, everyone grieves differently, so it's crucial to be kind to yourself and honor your own needs during this time.

C. Celebrating And Grieving At Christmas

C.1 Can I still celebrate holidays while grieving?

Absolutely! It is important to remember that grief does not mean you have to completely forego holiday celebrations. You can still participate in festivities while honoring your emotions and the memory of your loved one. Finding a balance between acknowledging your grief and engaging in holiday traditions can help you find moments of joy and healing during this time.

C.2 How do I cope with the conflicting emotions of grief and celebration?

It is important to acknowledge and validate your emotions. Allow yourself to feel the pain of grief while also recognizing that it is okay to experience moments of joy. Creating a safe space to process your emotions and seeking support from understanding individuals can help navigate these conflicting emotions.

C.3 How can I handle the pressure of family expectations during holidays?

Family expectations can add an additional layer of stress when grieving during the holidays. It is crucial to communicate openly with your family members about your feelings and needs. Setting realistic expectations and boundaries can help alleviate some of the pressure. Remember that it is okay to prioritize your well-being and adjust holiday plans to suit your emotional needs.

C.4 Should I attend holiday gatherings if I'm not feeling up to it?

Attending holiday gatherings is entirely up to you and how you are feeling. It is essential to listen to your intuition and give yourself permission to decline invitations or leave early if it becomes overwhelming. Communicate your needs to your loved ones, so they understand and respect your decision. Alternatively, you may choose to attend smaller, more intimate gatherings where you feel more comfortable and supported.

C.5 How can I honor and include the memory of my loved one during the holidays?

There are various ways to honor and include the memory of your loved one during the holidays. You can create a special remembrance ritual or dedicate a specific portion of your celebrations to share stories and memories. Hanging a stocking, lighting a candle, or displaying a photo of your loved one can serve as meaningful symbols of remembrance. Find what feels authentic to you and incorporate it into your holiday traditions as a way to keep their memory alive.

C.6 What are some self-care techniques that can help during celebratory times?
Engaging in activities that bring you comfort and solace can be beneficial. This might include spending time in nature, practicing mindfulness or meditation, journaling, engaging in creative outlets, or seeking out professional therapy or counseling. Prioritizing self-care allows you to nurture your emotional well-being amidst the celebrations.

D. Therapy And Coping With The Holiday Challenges

D.1 Is therapy during the holiday season effective?

Therapy during the holiday season can be highly effective. It provides a supportive and nonjudgmental space to explore and address the unique challenges that arise during this time. Therapists offer guidance, coping strategies, and a listening ear to help individuals navigate stress, grief, and other emotions that may intensify during the holidays.

D.2 How do I know if therapy is right for me during the holidays?

If you find yourself feeling overwhelmed, anxious, or struggling with the holiday season, therapy can be a beneficial option. It is particularly helpful if you experience holiday-related stress, grief, or loneliness. Consulting with a therapist can help determine if therapy is the right fit for your specific needs and goals during the holiday season.

D.3 What types of therapy are available for holiday-related challenges?

There are various types of therapy available to address holiday-related challenges. Individual therapy offers personalized support, while group therapy provides a sense of community and shared experiences. Family therapy can help improve communication and strengthen relationships during the holiday season. It's important to explore different therapy approaches and find the one that resonates with your specific needs and preferences.

D.4 How long should therapy continue during the holiday season?

The duration of therapy during the holiday season varies depending on individual circumstances. Some individuals may find short-term therapy helpful for immediate support and coping strategies, while others may benefit from longer-term therapy to address deeper issues. Discussing your goals and concerns with a therapist can help determine an appropriate timeline for your therapy journey during the holiday season.

Other Books/Ebooks In The (Eulogies: From Grieving To Healing Series)

Eulogies When Accidental Death Takes Our Beloved: Writing Guidelines, Examples and Templates (ISBN-13: 978-1-960176-16-5)

Eulogies When Long-Term Illness Takes Our Beloved: Writing Guidelines, Examples and Templates (ISBN-13: 978-1-960176-15-8)

Eulogies For Those We Lost To Sudden Illness: Writing Guidelines, Examples, and Templates (ISBN-13: 978-1-960176-14-1)